NUTRITION FOR WEIGHT LOSS SURGERY

Meal Plans

JUSTINE HAWKE & SALLY JOHNSTON

ACCREDITED PRACTISING DIETITIANS | ACCREDITED NUTRITIONISTS

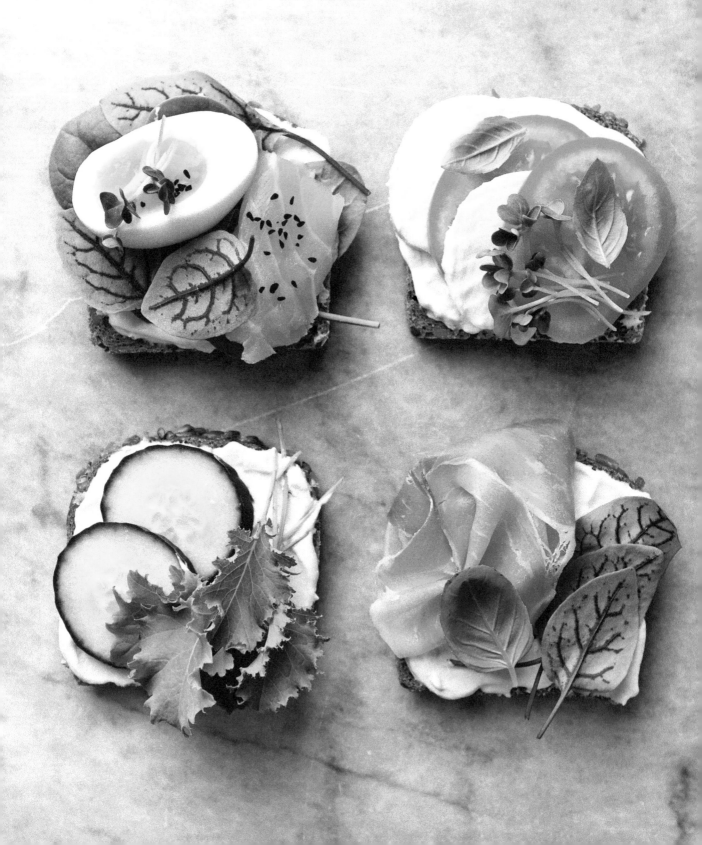

People often ask us, "What exactly should I be eating after weight loss surgery?"
It is a simple question, but not such a simple answer!

Whether you have had weight loss surgery or not, there is no one diet that suits everyone. Have you ever gone on a diet with your friend, relative or partner and lost a different amount of weight than they have? That is your body telling you that we are all different. So rather than a one size fits all approach, we have developed a framework to help you learn what is right for you and how to formulate a plan to suit **you**.

For those of you who track your food intake using smartphone apps, the following will interest you. (For those avoid the nitty gritty, you can tune out for a moment!) We tend to base our eating plans on the following balance:

- 30-35% of your total energy from protein

- 30% of your total energy from fat

- 35-40% of your total energy from carbohydrate, preferably low glycemic index (low GI) wherever possible.

This balance is not high protein, high carbohydrate or high fat. It isn't Keto, Paleo, Intermittent Fasting, 5:2, Atkins, Banting, Weight Watchers or Liver Cleansing. It is basic, simple stuff that serves most people well long term. It is not sexy or extreme like the diets and plans online or in magazines that go in and out of fashion. However, in our work with weight loss surgery clients, it is something we have found most people can eat comfortably, **long term** to help them lose weight and most importantly, **maintain that lost weight**.

We know that for many people to lose weight they must reduce the amount of food they eat and indeed this is the purpose of weight loss surgery. However, studies also tell us that reducing our energy intake below 800 calories (3,400 kilojoules) is **not** likely to be beneficial. In fact, it may be detrimental to weight management. The lowest energy intake we would ever recommend to a client would be 800 calories. You will therefore see our meal plans start at 800 calories (3,300 kilojoules) and range to 1,500 calories (6,200 kilojoules) per day.

Females, people who do little activity and those with a small capacity for food following surgery may only need 800 or 1,000 calories per day. Men, people who are more physically active, people in physically active jobs or those who have a larger capacity may need closer to 1,500 calories per day. Many people will need somewhere in between. The important thing to remember is that however many calories it may be, the balance of foods within that calorie level is important. That is what our meal plans aim to help with.

THE FOOD GROUPS

We use basic, simple food from all of the food groups in our meal plans.

To make this book easier to read however, we have shortened the names of the food groups.

Please note these terms will be used to refer to each of the food groups throughout this book:

GRAINS = breads, cereals, rice, pasta, noodles and starchy vegetables
FRUIT = fruit, dried fruit and juice
VEG = non starchy vegetables
MILK = milk and milk products
PROTEIN = meat and meat alternatives
FATS = fats and oils
EXTRAS = extras, indulgences and alcohol
FLAVOUR = flavour and moisture

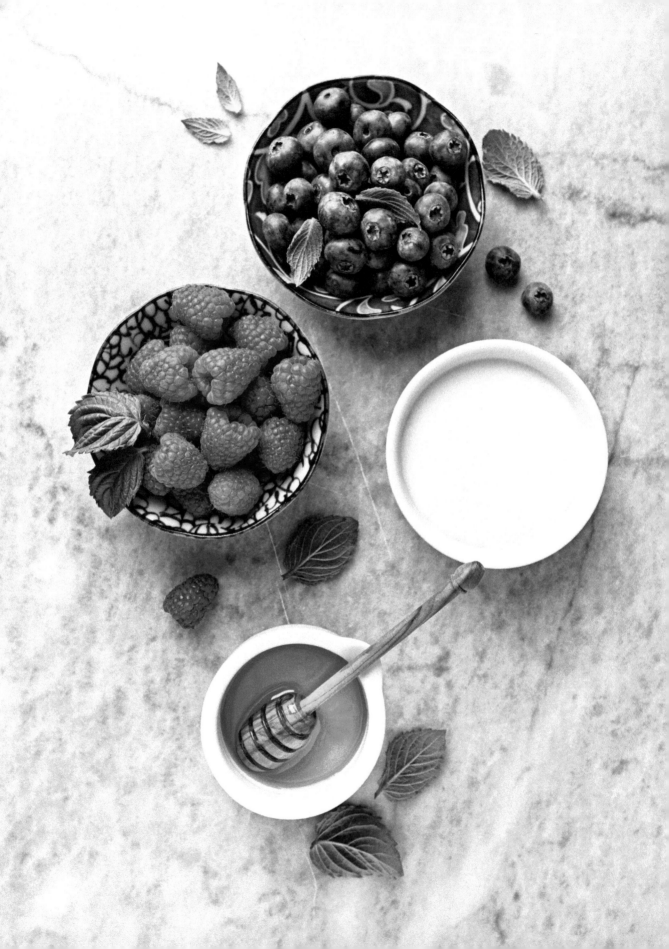

Guidelines for using the meal plans

The meal plans are intended as a **guideline**. You can follow them closely, or simply use them for inspiration and meal ideas. They are totally flexible.

The plans include four to six small meals and snacks each day, you may wish to eat more or less often – listen to your hunger and fullness signals and be guided by these. Ensure you also adjust your plan to suit your food tolerance, capacity and preferences using the food lists (page 11) provided (see *Adjusting Your Menu* below).

Some of the meal ideas are simple, one serve recipes, however can be increased to prepare multiple meals (for your family, or to freeze), such as mini meat loaves, rice muffins, chicken patties, etc.

It is important to keep hydrated by selecting suitable fluids from the *Food List (page 11)*. Aim for one and a half litres (1,500ml) daily as a minimum.

ADJUSTING YOUR MENU

The *Food Lists* provided give flexibility to adjust your meal plan to suit your individual needs. If you have specific foods you are unable to eat, or prefer not to eat, you can choose an alternative from the same food group. For example, if a meal includes bread and you are unable to tolerate bread, refer to the GRAINS list to see what you could have instead of bread. All of the foods listed in each group can be swapped, so you could swap 1 slice of bread for 1 wrap **or** 4 small Vita-Weat **or** ½ cup kidney beans, etc.

Examples of how you can change your meal plan are as follows:

- If you don't like the idea of having seven different breakfasts or lunches over a week, pick your favourite one or two and repeat these each day.

- If you are unable to tolerate a particular protein containing food such as red meat or chicken, you can select an alternative from the PROTEIN list that you are able to tolerate, such as fish or eggs.

- If you require a gluten free diet, select a gluten free alternative from the GRAINS list in place of gluten containing products.

- If you prefer to avoid all processed foods and a commercial product is listed (such as salsa, teriyaki marinade, etc.) you can leave it out or make your own.

- If you dislike a flavour combination or selected FLAVOUR suggestion you can select an alternative from the FLAVOUR list.

- If you are not hungry between meals, you may not need the snacks. However, if you find you are ravenous by the next meal and eat too quickly, the snacks may be useful to prevent you from getting over hungry. If you don't need these snacks, you can use these foods to make your meals a little larger if that suits you better.

EXTRAS

EXTRAS have an important role in healthy eating; they provide pleasure, they are social and add to quality of life. When they are included in small quantities, EXTRAS can help you stay on track by ensuring you do not feel deprived. It is not expected that you will **never** include these foods. All foods can have a place in your diet and no food should ever feel forbidden. However, quite simply, the more often you include these foods, the harder it is to manage your weight.

Aim to include no more than two to three EXTRAS per week. If your current intake is well in excess of this level, start by halving what you are currently having and work down towards the weekly goal of less than two to three. It really depends on where you are at in your journey. If you include these things on a regular basis, for example, more than twice a week and are not losing weight as you would like, then you need to look at changing this.

Alcohol is also high in energy and a regular intake can inhibit weight loss. For general health, it is recommended that we limit alcohol to no more than two standard drinks per day, with two alcohol free days per week. If you include alcohol regularly, even if it fits within these guidelines and are not losing as much weight as you would like, then you may need to adjust this.

PROTEIN

Protein is always a hot topic following weight loss surgery. If you follow our meal plans, you will also meet your minimum protein needs (60g per day). The **approximate** protein content of each meal plan is as follows:

- 800 calories: 60g protein per day

- 1,000 calories: 80-85g protein per day

- 1,200 calories: 90g protein per day

- 1,500 calories: 105g protein per day.

VITAMINS AND MINERALS

Whilst the plans are as nutritionally balanced as possible, they are less than most people eat and do not contain adequate micronutrients without vitamin and mineral supplements. Ensure you are including daily vitamin and mineral supplements that fits with your surgery type and individual needs, as guided by your health care team. Regular blood tests and appropriate vitamin and mineral supplementation are essential following weight loss surgery.

Which meal plan do I try first?

Not sure which meal plan you are best to start with? To get an idea of which meal plan may suit you, it is useful to use the checklist on the following page to see what your eating pattern looks like now.

Use the *Food Diary & Checklist* on page 6 to record what you eat for a few days. The more days you record your intake, the better picture you will get. We suggest two week days and one weekend day.

With each of the meals and snacks, use the checklist to work out roughly how many serves you think you are eating from each food group. Look carefully at the serve sizes on the food checklist to estimate your serve size – some foods are easy to eat more of than we think! It may be that you need to measure your serves to get a clear picture of what you are eating.

Once you have a record, add up the total amount of serves you have eaten in each food group each day. Average them out over how many days you kept the record. Enter your result in the table below.

FOOD GROUP	NO. OF SERVES I EAT PER DAY
GRAINS	
VEG	
FRUIT	
MILK	
PROTEIN	
FATS	
EXTRAS	

Now you can use the table to work out where you need to make changes to what you are eating.

Are you eating less that the number of serves in the 1,000 calorie plan and not losing weight, but would like to be? Then maybe you need to increase your intake to 1,000 calories. (If this does not help, you may need to see a dietitian who specialises in weight loss surgery for individualised advice.)

If you are eating close to the 1,500 calorie plan and not losing weight do not drop straight to the 1,000 calorie plan, you may only need to drop a couple of serves of food to find a level right for you.

Are you eating close to the 1,000 or 1,200 calorie plans but finding you are losing weight too quickly? Then maybe you need to increase your intake closer to the 1,500 calorie plan.

Did you find there were lots of foods in your diet that you were not sure how to categorise into food groups? Are they are actually 'extra' foods and hindering your weight loss progress?

This activity is just designed to get you thinking about where you are and how to move forward.

Food Diary & Checklist

MEAL OR SNACK	FOOD EATEN	SERVES EATEN FROM EACH FOOD GROUP	
Breakfast		PROTEIN	
		VEG	
		FRUIT	
		MILK	
		PROTEIN	
		FATS	
		EXTRAS	
Mid Morning		PROTEIN	
		VEG	
		FRUIT	
		MILK	
		PROTEIN	
		FATS	
		EXTRAS	
Lunch		PROTEIN	
		VEG	
		FRUIT	
		MILK	
		PROTEIN	
		FATS	
		EXTRAS	
Mid Afternoon		PROTEIN	
		VEG	
		FRUIT	
		MILK	
		PROTEIN	
		FATS	
		EXTRAS	
Dinner		PROTEIN	
		VEG	
		FRUIT	
		MILK	
		PROTEIN	
		FATS	
		EXTRAS	
Supper		PROTEIN	
		VEG	
		FRUIT	
		MILK	
		PROTEIN	
		FATS	
		EXTRAS	

Meal Plan Structure

Once you have an idea of which meal plan you would like to start with, you may like to prepare your food lists (page 8) so that you can vary the plan to suit yourself. (Alternatively you can jump straight to the plan and worry about the food lists only if you need them – it's completely up to you!)

The table below tells you how many serves from each food group you can use in each of the meal plans. You will see on the food lists there is a space to write in how many serves you can choose each day. This will help you vary your meal plan if you want to.

	800 CALORIES (3,300 KILOJOULES)	1,000 CALORIES (4,200 KILOJOULES)	1,200 CALORIES (5,000 KILOJOULES)	1,500 CALORIES (6,300 KILOJOULES)
GRAINS*	2	3	4	5
MILK	2	2 - 2½	2-3	3
VEG	Unlimited as tolerated	Unlimited as tolerated	Unlimited as tolerated	Unlimited as tolerated
FRUIT*	1	1	1	2
PROTEIN	1	1½ – 2	1½ – 2	2
FATS	2	2	3	4
EXTRAS	Maximum 2 – 3 per week			
FLAVOUR	Use in small amounts as needed.			
FLUID	Aim for 1.5L per day			

*If you would prefer to eat less breads, cereals and starchy vegetable, you can replace one of these serves with a serve of fruit.

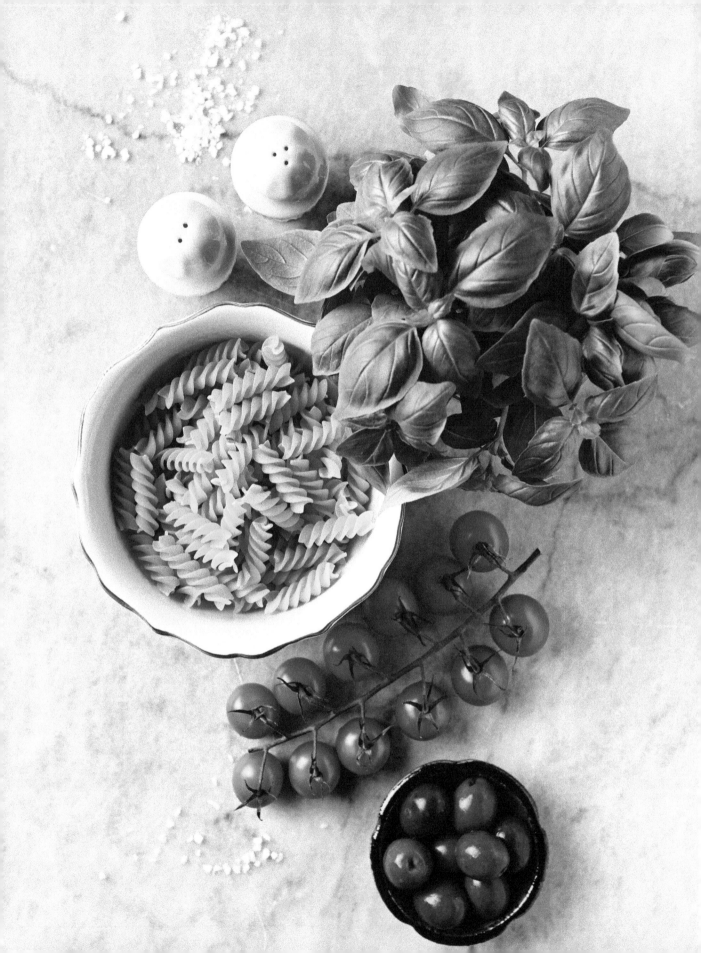

Food Lists

GRAINS

(BREADS, CEREALS, RICE, PASTA, NOODLES AND STARCHY VEGETABLES)

Each serve provides approximately 15-20g of carbohydrate.

1 serve is approximately:

- 1 slice bread or ½ medium sized bread roll (wholegrain)
- ½ small or ¼ large pita/pocket bread
- 1 wrap (if less than 20g carbohydrate per wrap)
- 1 crumpet
- 1 slice fruit loaf or raisin bread
- ½ English muffin
- ½ cup All-Bran or Bran Flakes
- ¾ cup cooked porridge (¼ cup raw oats)
- ¼ cup natural muesli
- approx ½ cup (30-40g) cereal eg. Sultana Bran, Uncle Tobys Plus Mix
- 1½ Weet-Bix or Vita Brits
- ½ cup cooked pasta or wheat noodles
- 50g cooked gnocchi
- ½ cup cooked quinoa
- ½ cup cooked buckwheat
- ½ cup cooked cornmeal
- 2 tablespoon breadcrumbs
- 1 lasagne sheet
- 1/3 cup cooked basmati/Doongara/Mahatma/brown rice, rice noodles, barley or couscous
- 2 rice paper sheets or 3 wonton wrappers
- 6 small squares Salada or Premium crackers(preferably wholemeal/grain)
- 2 sandwich size or 4 small Vita-Weat
- 3 Ryvita
- 3 cups air popped popcorn
- ½ cup pretzels
- 2 tablespoons flour
- 1 medium potato or ½ cup mashed potato
- 1 small or ½ large sweet potato
- 1 medium swede
- ½ large cob or ½ cup sweet corn
- 1½ cups broad beans
- 1 cup cooked split peas
- ½ cup baked beans, 3 bean mix, chick peas and kidney beans
- ¾ cup lentils.

Note: Wholemeal or wholegrain products are the best choices.

MILK

Each serve provides approximately 10g of protein and 300mg of calcium.

1 serve is approximately:

- 250mL milk , soy milk or high protein milk eg. The Complete Dairy

- 200g yoghurt (with little added sugar)

- 2 slices of cheese (approx 40g)

- 120g (½ cup) ricotta cheese

- 120g (½ cup) cottage cheese.

Note: Low or reduced fat varieties help reduce your energy intake and should be chosen if weight reduction is your main priority. High protein options such as Chobani™ yoghurts, YoPRO yoghurts and Complete Dairy High Protein milks are also useful to help you meet your protein targets. Ricotta and cottage cheese are lower in calcium and should not be used as your main source of calcium.

VEG

Two to three serves per day are recommended, however you can include more, particularly if you have a larger capacity and/or are hungry on the recommended amount of food. The health benefits of eating additional non starchy vegetables far outweighs any additional calories or kilojoules they may add to your diet.

1 serve is ½ a cup of cooked vegetables or 1 cup of salad vegetables from the following:

- alfalfa sprouts
- artichokes
- bamboo shoots
- bean sprouts
- beetroot
- broccoli
- brussell sprouts
- cabbage
- capsicum
- carrots
- cauliflower
- celery
- chives
- choko
- cucumber
- eggplant
- endives
- fennel
- garlic
- green beans
- lettuce

- leeks
- marrow
- mushrooms
- cress
- onions
- parsley
- parsnip
- peas
- silverbeet
- spring onions
- squash
- snow peas
- sauerkraut
- sprouts
- tomatoes
- turnips
- watercress
- water chestnuts
- zucchini
- radishes
- shallots.

FRUIT

(FRUIT, DRIED FRUIT AND FRUIT JUICE)

Each serve provides approximately 15g of carbohydrate.

1 serve is approximately:

- 1 average pear, banana, apple, orange or peach

- 2-3 apricots, plums, kiwi fruit, mandarins or nectarines

- ½ mango

- 20 medium grapes

- 2 cups diced rockmelon or watermelon

- 1 cup diced honeydew melon or diced pineapple

- ¾ cup canned fruit in natural juice (drained) eg. apricots, peaches

- 1½ tablespoons sultanas

- 30g dried fruit

- 4 dried apple rings

- 2 dried pear halves

- ½ cup (125mL) orange, apple or pineapple juice

- 1½ cups vegetable or tomato juice

- 1 punnet strawberries

- 1 cup blueberries, raspberries, blackberries.

Note: Eat rhubarb, passionfruit, strawberries, lime, lemon & loquats freely. Limit juices and choose whole fruit where possible.

PROTEIN

Meat and meat alternatives vary in the amount of protein they provide.

The following provide approx 25g protein per serve.

One serve is approximately:

- 100g raw lean meat eg. steak, 2 small lamb chops, 2 slices roast meat

- 1/2 cup lean mince

- 100g raw (1/2 small) chicken with skin removed

- 120g raw fish and seafood

- 100g canned fish

- 150g tempeh

- 150g quorn

- 1/4 cup savoury yeast flakes.

The following provide approx 20g protein per serve.

One serve is approximately:

- 3/4 cup cooked lentils

- 1/2 cup edamame

- 100g tofu.

The following provide approx 10-15g protein per serve.

One serve is approximately:

- 2 eggs

- 1 cup canned or cooked legumes eg. chickpeas, kidney beans, baked beans, etc.

FATS

(FATS)

Each serve provides approximately 5g of fat.

1 serve is approximately:

- 1 teaspoon of margarine

- 1 teaspoon oil eg. olive, canola, sunflower, coconut

- 25g avocado (approximately 1/8 of an avocado)

- 10g nuts (approx 7-8 cashews or almonds, 3 walnuts or brazil nuts)

- 10g (2 teaspoons) nut paste eg. almond, peanut

- 10g seeds eg. flaxseed, chia, sunflower

- 10g tahini.

FLAVOUR

USE FREELY:

- herbs and spices
- curry powder
- low fat/fat free mayonnaise and dressings
- vinegars (balsamic, apple cider, red wine, white wine, etc.)
- reduced salt stock.

USE IN SMALL AMOUNTS AS NEEDED:

- mayonnaise and dressings
- pickles
- chutney
- relish
- hommous
- tzatziki
- Philadelphia Extra Light cream cheese
- gherkins
- olives
- capers
- pickled onion
- chargrilled peppers (capsicums)
- other pickled vegetables (avoiding those picked in oil)
- salt reduced soy sauce
- hoisin, oyster, sweet chili, tomato and barbeque sauces.

FLUIDS

AIM FOR A MINIMUM OF 1.5 LITRES PER DAY:

- water
- herbal tea
- soda water (if tolerated)
- diet/sugar free cordial
- tea and coffee (with a small dash of low fat milk)
- clear protein waters such as Protein Perfection and BODIE'z.

EXTRAS

1 serve is approximately:

- 1 small slice (40g) cake or doughnut

- 2 chocolate or cream filled biscuits

- 30g chocolate

- 1 small bag (30g) potato crisps

- 2 tablespoons (35g) pate

- 2 thin slices (30g) processed meat e.g. salami

- 1/3 meat pie, pasty or sausage roll

- ½ slice large pizza

- 10 (40g) hot chips

- 40g hard or 50g soft lollies

- 2 small glasses wine

- 1 pint full strength beer

- 2 stubbies light beer

- 2 single pours of spirits

- 1 ½ single pours of liqueur.

Note: Include 2 alcohol free days per week. Those with particular medical conditions may need to limit further.

Create Your Own Menu

MEAL OR SNACK	SERVES FROM EACH FOOD GROUP		MEAL AND SNACK IDEAS
Breakfast	GRAINS		
	VEG		
	FRUIT		
	MILK		
	PROTEIN		
	FATS		
	EXTRAS		
Morning Tea	GRAINS		
	VEG		
	FRUIT		
	MILK		
	PROTEIN		
	FATS		
	EXTRAS		
Lunch	GRAINS		
	VEG		
	FRUIT		
	MILK		
	PROTEIN		
	FATS		
	EXTRAS		
Afternoon Tea	GRAINS		
	VEG		
	FRUIT		
	MILK		
	PROTEIN		
	FATS		
	EXTRAS		
Dinner	GRAINS		
	VEG		
	FRUIT		
	MILK		
	PROTEIN		
	FATS		
	EXTRAS		
Supper	GRAINS		
	VEG		
	FRUIT		
	MILK		
	PROTEIN		
	FATS		
	EXTRAS		

Meal Plans

....

800 Calorie Meal Plan: Day 1

MEAL	FOOD GROUP	SERVE/S	FOOD CHOICE	MEAL IDEA
Breakfast	GRAINS	½	1 Weet-Bix	Weet-Bix with milk and sliced banana.
	MILK	½	125ml milk	
	FRUIT	½	½ small banana	
Mid Morning	MILK	½	100g yoghurt	Yoghurt
Lunch	GRAINS	1	2 small Vita-Weat	Vita-Weat with cheese, sliced tomato and pickles.
	MILK	1	2 slices cheese	
	VEG		Sliced tomato	
	FLAVOUR		Pickles	
Mid Afternoon	FATS	1	10g unsalted, dry roasted or raw nuts.	Fruit and nut mix.
	FRUIT	½	10 grapes	
Dinner	PROTEIN	1	100g chicken	Honey, soy and garlic chicken with Asian greens: Let chicken sit in marinade and then grill in olive oil. Serve with steamed Asian greens.
	FLAVOUR		Honey, soy and garlic marinade.	
	FATS	1	1 teaspoon olive oil	
	VEG		Asian green vegetables such as bok choy, broccollini, Chinese cabbage, etc.	
Evening Snack	GRAINS	½	½ cups air popped popcorn	Popcorn

800 Calorie Meal Plan: Day 2

MEAL	FOOD GROUP	SERVE/S	FOOD CHOICE	MEAL IDEA
Breakfast	GRAINS	½	2 tablespoons natural muesli	Muesli with yoghurt and mixed berries.
	MILK	½	100g yoghurt	
	FRUIT	½	½ cup mixed berries	
Mid Morning	FRUIT	½	½ kiwi fruit	Fruit
Lunch	PROTEIN	½	60g tuna in spring water	Mediterranean tuna salad wrap: Spread wrap bread with hummus or tzatziki. Top with drained tuna and diced vegetables before wrapping.
	GRAINS	½	½ wrap	
	VEG	½	Diced cucumber, tomato, red onion, and capsicum.	
	FLAVOUR		Hummus or tzatziki.	
Mid Afternoon	MILK	½	100g yoghurt	Yoghurt
Dinner	PROTEIN	½	50g lamb	**Spiced lamb salad:** Rub lamb in spices and olive oil and grill. Serve with salad of drained chickpeas, diced roasted sweet potato and other vegetables. Top with a dollop of Greek yoghurt mixed with coriander and lemon juice.
	FLAVOUR		Smoked paprika, ground cumin and coriander.	
	FATS	1	1 teaspoon olive oil	
	GRAINS	1	¼ cup chick peas and ½ small sweet potato, roasted and diced.	
	VEG		Diced cucumber, tomato and capsicum.	
	FLAVOUR		Greek yoghurt, coriander and lemon juice.	
Evening Snack	FATS	1	10g unsalted, dry roasted or raw nuts.	Nuts

800 Calorie Meal Plan: Day 3

MEAL	FOOD GROUP	SERVE/S	FOOD CHOICE	MEAL IDEA
Breakfast	GRAINS	½	½ wholemeal crumpet	Top crumpet with cheese and grill until cheese is melted.
	MILK	½	20g cheese	
Mid Morning	MILK	1	250ml milk	Milk drink eg. small latte, cappuccino or flat white OR 1 cup milk with 2 teaspoons Milo or low sugar, low fat flavoured milk.
Lunch	MEAT	½	¼ cup 4-bean mix	Mexican bean salad: Combine beans, corn, diced vegetables and shredded herbs. Mix, and top with lime juice and finely diced chilli.
	GRAINS	1	½ cup corn kernels	
	VEG		Diced tomato and capsicum, shredded coriander and mint.	
	FLAVOUR		Lime juice and chilli.	
Mid Afternoon	MILK	½	100g yoghurt	Fruit and yoghurt.
	FRUIT	½	½ apple	
Dinner	PROTEIN	½	50g lean pork mince	Chinese BBQ pork stir fry: Mix marinade through pork mince. Stir-fry with thinly sliced vegetables and serve with noodles.
	FLAVOUR		Chinese BBQ pork marinade	
	GRAINS	½	¼ cup noodles	
	VEG		Thinly sliced carrot, zucchini, red onion and capsicum.	
Evening Snack	FRUIT	½	½ punnet strawberries	Fruit

800 Calorie Meal Plan: Day 4

MEAL	FOOD GROUP	SERVE/S	FOOD CHOICE	MEAL IDEA
Breakfast	GRAINS	1	½ English muffin	Baked beans and cheese muffin: Top muffin with margarine, baked beans and cheese, grill until cheese has melted.
	GRAINS	½	¼ cup baked beans	
	MILK	½	1 slice cheese	
	FATS	1	1 teaspoon margarine	
Mid Morning	GRAINS	½	2 small Vita-Weat	Cheese and crackers
	MILK	½	1 slice cheese	
Lunch	PROTEIN	½	50g chicken, shredded	Chicken and vegetable soup: Cook vegetables, garlic and leek. Add salt reduced stock powder and shredded chicken. Flavour with preferred herbs and spices.
	VEG		Diced carrot, celery, zucchini and swede or turnip.	
	FLAVOUR		Salt reduced stock powder, leek, garlic, herbs and spices.	
Mid Afternoon	MILK	1	200g yoghurt	Fruit and yoghurt.
	FRUIT	½	¼ cup berries	
Dinner	PROTEIN	½	50g salmon	One pan oven baked salmon and vegetables: Combine vegetables and salmon in sheet pan, season with lemon juice, salt, and cracked black pepper. Bake.
	VEG		Zucchini, cherry tomatoes and broccoli.	
	FLAVOUR		Lemon juice, salt and cracked black pepper.	
Evening Snack	FRUIT	½	½ apple	Spread apple slices with nut butter.
	FATS	1	1 teaspoon peanut or almond butter	

800 Calorie Meal Plan: Day 5

MEAL	FOOD GROUP	SERVE/S	FOOD CHOICE	MEAL IDEA
Breakfast	GRAINS	1	1 slice wholegrain bread	Smashed avocado Mash avocado and spread on grainy toast. Top with squeeze of lime, chilli, salt and cracked black pepper.
	FATS	1	25g avocado	
	FLAVOUR		Lime, chilli, salt and cracked black pepper.	
Mid Morning	MILK	1	250ml milk	Milk drink eg. small latte, cappuccino or flat white OR 1 cup milk with 2 teaspoons Milo or low sugar, low fat flavoured milk.
Lunch	MILK	1	40g feta	Greek salad: Mix diced vegetables, olives and feta together. Top with lemon juice, oil and cracked black pepper.
	FATS	1	1 teaspoon olive oil	
	VEG		Diced cucumber, tomato and capsicum.	
	FLAVOUR		Lemon, cracked black pepper and black olives.	
Mid Afternoon	VEG		Celery, carrot and cucumber sticks.	Vegetable sticks and salsa.
	FLAVOUR		Tomato salsa.	
Dinner	PROTEIN	1	½ cup lean beef mince	Spaghetti Bolognese: Brown garlic, onion and beef mince. Add grated carrot, zucchini and canned tomato. Mix through basil, oregano, cooked pasta and serve with cracked black pepper.
	VEG		Diced onion, grated carrot and zucchini and tinned tomato.	
	FLAVOUR		Garlic, basil, oregano and cracked black pepper.	
	GRAINS	1	½ cup pasta	
Evening Snack	FRUIT		30g dried fruit	Dried fruit

800 Calorie Meal Plan: Day 6

MEAL	FOOD GROUP	SERVE/S	FOOD CHOICE	MEAL IDEA
Breakfast	MILK	1	250ml milk	Strawberry smoothie: Blend milk and strawberries until smooth.
	FRUIT	½	½ punnet strawberries	
Mid Morning	FATS	1	1 teaspoon peanut or almond paste	Celery sticks with nut paste.
Lunch	GRAINS	1	3 Ryvita crackers	Ryvitas and cheese: Spread Ryvitas with cottage cheese. Top with sliced tomato and pickles.
	MILK	½	¼ cup cottage cheese	
	VEG		Sliced tomato	
	FLAVOUR		Pickles	
Mid Afternoon	MILK	½	100g yoghurt	Fruit and yoghurt
	FRUIT	½	½ small banana	
Dinner	GRAINS	1	2 rice paper sheets	Chicken cold rolls: Prepare rice paper sheets as directed. Spread with sweet chilli sauce. Top with chicken and vegetables, roll.
	PROTEIN	1	½ small chicken breast, skin removed, steamed and shredded	
	VEG		Thinly sliced carrot, cucumber and capsicum.	
	FLAVOUR		Sweet chilli sauce	
Evening Snack	FATS	1	10g unsalted, dry roasted or raw nuts.	Nuts

800 Calorie Meal Plan: Day 7

MEAL	FOOD GROUP	SERVE/S	FOOD CHOICE	MEAL IDEA
Breakfast	GRAINS	1	¼ cup raw oats	Porridge: Cook oats in milk using preferred method.
	MILK	½	125ml milk	
Mid Morning	GRAINS	1	¼ cup pretzels	Pretzles
Lunch	PROTEIN	½	1 slice roast meat	Grazing plate: Prepare a plate of sliced roast meat, sliced cheese, nuts, vegetable sticks and dip.
	MILK	1	2 slices cheese	
	FATS	1	10g almonds	
	VEG		Celery, carrot and cucumber sticks.	
	FLAVOUR		Hummus and tzatziki.	
Mid Afternoon	FRUIT	½	½ pear	Fruit
Dinner	PROTEIN	½	60g raw fresh fish	Summer style fish: Grill fish in olive oil. Serve with salsa of diced mango, cucumber and tomato, and top with squeeze of lime and coriander.
	FATS	1	1 teaspoon olive oil	
	FRUIT	½	½ medium mango cheek	
	VEG		Cucumber and tomato.	
	FLAVOUR		Lime and coriander.	
Evening Snack	MILK	½	100g yoghurt	Yoghurt

1,000 Calorie Meal Plan: Day 1

MEAL	FOOD GROUP	SERVE/S	FOOD CHOICE	MEAL IDEA
Breakfast	GRAINS	½	2 tablespoons muesli	Small bowl yoghurt topped with blueberries and muesli.
	MILK	½	100g yoghurt	
	FRUIT	½	½ cup blueberries	
Mid Morning	GRAINS	½	2 Vita-Weat crackers	Vita-Weat with sliced cheese and relish.
	MILK	½	20g cheese	
	FLAVOUR		1 teaspoons relish	
Lunch	PROTEIN	1	120g tuna in spring water	Tuna salad wrap: Combine tuna with finely diced celery, diced gherkin, low fat mayonnaise and wholegrain mustard and add to wrap.
	GRAINS	1	1 wrap	
	VEG		Celery and gherkin.	
	FLAVOUR		Low fat mayonnaise and wholegrain mustard.	
Mid Afternoon	FATS	2	20g nuts	20g unsalted, dry roasted nuts
Dinner	PROTEIN	1	100g lamb	Moroccan lamb salad: Top baby spinach with grilled lamb, chickpeas and baked sweet potato and dress with Moroccan Dressing – see *Dressing Recipes* (page 51).
	GRAINS	1	¼ cup chickpeas ½ small sweet potato	
	VEG		Baby spinach	
Evening Snack	FRUIT	½	1 kiwi fruit	Dice fruit and eat as is with yoghurt, or blend yoghurt and fruit together and freeze in an ice block mold.
	MILK	1	200g yoghurt	

1,000 Calorie Meal Plan: Day 2

MEAL	FOOD GROUP	SERVE/S	FOOD CHOICE	MEAL IDEA
Breakfast	GRAINS	1	1 slice multigrain toast	Multigrain toast spread with avocado and topped with a poached egg.
	PROTEIN	½	1 egg	
	FATS	2	¼ avocado	
Mid Morning	FRUIT	1	Small bunch (approx. 20) grapes	Grapes
Lunch	GRAINS	1	4 Vita-Weat crackers	Vita-Weat crackers topped with cottage cheese, ham and sliced cucumber and/or tomato.
	MILK	½	¼ cup cottage cheese	
	PROTEIN	½	50g ham	
	VEG		Cucumber and/or tomato.	
Mid Afternoon	MILK	1	250ml milk	Small latte, cappuccino or flat white OR 1 cup milk with 2 teaspoons milo OR low sugar, low fat flavoured milk.
Dinner	PROTEIN	1	100g chicken mince	Chicken tacos: Cook mince, diced onion, kidney beans and salsa. Add to taco and top with shredded lettuce, grated carrot and diced tomato.
	GRAINS	½	¼ cup kidney beans 1 taco shell	
	VEG		Lettuce, carrot and tomato.	
	FLAVOUR		Salsa	
Evening Snack	GRAINS	½	1½ cups air popped popcorn	Small bowl air popped popcorn sprinkled with cinnamon. Milo or milk coffee (½ milk, ½ hot water) using 2 teaspoons Milo or coffee.
	MILK	½	125ml milk	
	FLAVOUR		Cinnamon	

1,000 Calorie Meal Plan: Day 3

MEAL	FOOD GROUP	SERVE/S	FOOD CHOICE	MEAL IDEA
Breakfast	GRAINS	1	1½ Weet-Bix	Weet-Bix with milk and sliced banana.
	MILK	½	125ml milk	
	FRUIT	1	Small banana	
Mid Morning				
Lunch	GRAINS	1	1 slice multigrain bread	Vegetable, chicken and lentil soup: Use a powdered, salt reduced stock base, add vegetables from non-starchy vegetables list, shredded chicken and lentils.
	PROTEIN	1	50g chicken tenderloin ½ cup lentils	
	FATS	1	1 teaspoon margarine	Serve with 1 slice multigrain toast with a scrape of margarine.
	VEG		Non starchy vegetables/ salad of your choice.	
Mid Afternoon	MILK	1	200g yoghurt	Yoghurt
Dinner	PROTEIN	1	100g lean steak	Meat and vegetables: Marinated steak (cut across the grain in thin slices, chew well) with cheesy mashed potato, gravy and steamed non-starchy vegetables from list.
	GRAINS	1	½ cup mashed potato	
	MILK	½	20g cheese	
	FATS	1	1 teaspoon margarine	
	VEG		Non starchy vegetables/ salad of your choice.	
Evening Snack				

1,000 Calorie Meal Plan: Day 4

MEAL	FOOD GROUP	SERVE/S	FOOD CHOICE	MEAL IDEA
Breakfast	GRAINS	1	¼ cup rolled oats	Porridge
	MILK	½	125ml milk	
Mid Morning	MILK	1	250ml milk	Small latte, cappuccino or flat white OR 1 cup milk with 2 teaspoons milo OR low sugar, low fat flavoured milk.
Lunch	GRAINS	2	1 English muffin	English muffin spread with tomato relish and topped with scrambled eggs.
	PROTEIN	1	2 eggs	
	FLAVOUR		1 teaspoon tomato relish	
Mid Afternoon	FATS	2	20g (1 tablespoon) nut paste eg. almond or peanut	Spread celery (if tolerated, strings removed) or carrot sticks with nut paste.
	VEG		Celery and carrot sticks.	
Dinner	PROTEIN	1	120g salmon fillet	Baked Salmon with Asian Greens: Wrap salmon in foil and bake in the oven. Serve with steamed Asian green vegetables with garlic, lemon and oyster sauce.
	VEG		Asian green vegetables such as bok choy, broccollini, Chinese cabbage, etc.	
	FLAVOUR		1 teaspoon Oyster sauce, garlic and lemon juice	
Evening Snack	FRUIT	1	1 apple	Baked apple with yoghurt (peel apple if you do not tolerate the skin).
	MILK	½	¼ cup yoghurt	

1,000 Calorie Meal Plan: Day 5

MEAL	FOOD GROUP	SERVE/S	FOOD CHOICE	MEAL IDEA
Breakfast	GRAINS	1	1 slice multigrain bread	Baked beans and avocado on toast.
	PROTEIN	1	½ cup baked beans	
	FATS	2	¼ avocado	
Mid Morning	MILK	1	250ml milk	Small latte, cappuccino or flat white OR 1 cup milk with 2 teaspoons milo OR low sugar, low fat flavoured milk.
Lunch	GRAINS	1	½ English Muffin	Mini pizza: Top English muffin with tomato paste, finely diced mushroom, tomato, basil and cheese. Grill until cheese is melted.
	MILK	½	20g cheese	
	VEG		Mushroom, tomato and basil.	
	FLAVOUR		Tomato paste	
Mid Afternoon	FRUIT	1	½ cup tinned fruit in natural juice	Tinned fruit
Dinner	PROTEIN	½	50g chicken	Chicken wrap: Shred a BBQ chicken breast, combine with a handful of salad leaves and low fat mayonnaise in a wrap.
	GRAINS	1	1 wrap	
	VEG		Mixed salad leaves	
	FLAVOUR		Low fat mayonnaise	
Evening Snack	MILK	1	200g yoghurt	Yoghurt

1,000 Calorie Meal Plan: Day 6

MEAL	FOOD GROUP	SERVE/S	FOOD CHOICE	MEAL IDEA
Breakfast	GRAINS	1	1 wholemeal crumpet	Crumpet with cheese and vegemite.
	MILK	½	20g cheese	
	FATS	1	1 teaspoon margarine	
Mid Morning	GRAINS	½	6 small rice cracker biscuits	Crackers with dried fruit and nuts.
	FRUIT	1	5 dried apricots (10 halves)	
	FATS	1	10g nuts eg. almonds, cashews, walnuts	
Lunch	GRAINS	½	¼ cup sweet corn kernels	Sweet corn and bean salad: Combine corn kernels, bean mix, blanched green beans and grated red onion. Dress with vinegar based dressing – see dressing recipes attached.
	PROTEIN	½	½ cup five bean mix	
	VEG		Green beans and red onion.	
Mid Afternoon	MILK	1	200g yoghurt	1 tub yoghurt
Dinner	PROTEIN	1	100g lean pork mince	Pork meatballs: Combine pork mince, relish, grated onion and a lightly beaten egg to roll into balls. Serve with couscous and steamed vegetables.
	GRAINS	1	1/3 cup cooked couscous	
	FLAVOUR		2 tablespoons tomato relish	
	VEG		Non starchy vegetables of your choice.	
Evening Snack	MILK	1	250ml milk	Small latte, cappuccino or flat white OR 1 cup milk with 2 teaspoons milo OR low sugar, low fat flavoured milk.

1,000 Calorie Meal Plan: Day 7

MEAL	FOOD GROUP	SERVE/S	FOOD CHOICE	MEAL IDEA
Breakfast	MILK	1	200ml milk 50g yoghurt	Breakfast smoothie: Blend all ingredients together. If you like a green smoothie, add spinach or kale.
	FRUIT	1	½ cup frozen berries ½ frozen banana	
	FATS	1	1 teaspoon ground seeds eg. LSA	
	VEG		Non starchy vegetables/ salad	
Mid Morning				
Lunch	GRAINS	1	1 wrap	Spread wrap with small amount of relish or chutney, top with ham, avocado and salad.
	PROTEIN	½	50g shaved ham	
	VEG		Non starchy salad of your choice.	
	FATS	1	1/8 avocado	
	FLAVOUR		1 teaspoon relish or chutney	
Mid Afternoon	PROTEIN	1	100g tuna	Tuna with carrot and celery sticks.
	VEG		Non starchy vegetables/ salad	
Dinner	MILK	1	¼ cup ricotta cheese ¼ cup cottage cheese	Spinach and ricotta cannelloni: Combine cheeses with frozen, chopped spinach (squeeze out excess moisture) and nutmeg. Fill cannelloni tubes, pour tomato passata over the top and bake.
	GRAINS	1	1½ cannelloni tubes	
	VEG		Spinach and tomato passata (tomato puree/ sauce).	
Evening Snack	GRAINS	1	4 Vita-Weat crackers	Cheese and crackers.
	MILK	½	20g cheese	

1,200 Calorie Meal Plan: Day 1

MEAL	FOOD GROUP	SERVE/S	FOOD CHOICE	MEAL IDEA
Breakfast	GRAINS	2	2 slices raisin bread	Raisin toast
	FATS	1	1 teaspoon margarine	
Mid Morning	MILK	1	200g yoghurt	Yoghurt
Lunch	GRAINS	1	Small potato	Microwaved jacket potato topped with baked beans and grated cheese.
	PROTEIN	½	½ cup baked beans	
	MILK	½	20g grated cheese	
Mid Afternoon	FATS	2	20g almonds	Small handful almonds and dried apricots.
	FRUIT	½	5 dried apricot halves	
Dinner	PROTEIN	1	120g cooked salmon	Salmon and caper wrap: Spread wrap with cream cheese and relish. Top with salmon, capers and salad leaves. Add diced tomato if desired.
	GRAINS	1	1 wrap	
	VEG		Salad leaves	
	FLAVOUR		1 teaspoon capers 1 teaspoon low fat cream cheese 1 teaspoon tomato relish	
Evening Snack	FRUIT	½	Diced watermelon (up to 1 cup)	Fruit plus milk drink eg. Small latte, cappuccino or flat white OR 1 cup milk with 2 teaspoons milo OR low sugar, low fat flavoured milk.
	MILK	1	250ml milk drink	

1,200 Calorie Meal Plan: Day 2

MEAL	FOOD GROUP	SERVE/S	FOOD CHOICE	MEAL IDEA
Breakfast	GRAINS	1	1 slice grainy toast	Toast topped with scrambled eggs and grated cheese.
	MILK	1	40g cheese	
	PROTEIN	1	2 eggs	
Mid Morning				
Lunch	GRAINS	1	½ cup cooked quinoa	Feta, walnut and beetroot salad with quinoa: Combine quinoa, diced beetroot, crumbled feta and walnuts with rocket leaves. Dress with balsamic vinegar and olive oil.
	MILK	1	40g feta	
	FATS	3	20g walnuts plus 1 teaspoon olive oil	
	VEG	1	Beetroot and rocket leaves.	
	FLAVOUR		Balsamic vinegar	
Mid Afternoon	GRAINS	1	4 Vita-Weat crackers	Vita-Weat crackers with hommus.
	FLAVOUR		2 teaspoons hommus	
Dinner	PROTEIN	1	100g chicken mince	Mexican inspired chicken mince: Cook onion and chicken mince in a frying pan. Add kidney beans, frozen peas and spinach then pour over salsa.
	GRAINS	1	½ cup kidney beans	
	VEG	1	Onion, frozen peas and spinach.	
	FLAVOUR		Salsa	
Evening Snack	FRUIT	1	Strawberries (up to 1 punnet)	Strawberries and yoghurt.
	MILK	1	200g yoghurt	

1,200 Calorie Meal Plan: Day 3

MEAL	FOOD GROUP	SERVE/S	FOOD CHOICE	MEAL IDEA
Breakfast	GRAINS	1	½ cup untoasted muesli	Muesli and milk.
	MILK	½	125ml milk	
Mid Morning	FATS	3	30g unsalted mixed nuts and seeds.	Nuts and seeds.
Lunch	GRAINS	1	1 wrap	Tuna and salad wrap: Top wrap with tuna, baby spinach, tomato, red onion and a squeeze of lemon. Add low fat mayo.
	PROTEIN	1	120g tinned tuna in spring water	
	VEG		Baby spinach, tomato and red onion.	
	FLAVOUR		Low fat mayo	
Mid Afternoon	FRUIT	1	Small bunch (20) grapes	Fruit and yoghurt.
	MILK	1	200g yoghurt	
Dinner	PROTEIN	1	½ cup beef mince Egg to combine	Open home-made hamburgers: Combine mince, egg, grated onion, herbs and spices. Shape into patties and grill. Top roll with relish, salad, cheese and patty.
	GRAINS	2	½ small grainy roll	
	VEG		Non starchy salad of your choice eg. lettuce, tomato, cucumber or carrot.	
	MILK	½	20g cheese	
	FLAVOUR		1 teaspoon relish or chutney	
Evening Snack				

1,200 Calorie Meal Plan: Day 4

MEAL	FOOD GROUP	SERVE/S	FOOD CHOICE	MEAL IDEA
Breakfast	GRAINS	1	¼ cup oats	Porridge topped with cinnamon and sultanas.
	MILK	1	250 ml milk	
	FRUIT	1	1½ tablespoons sultanas	
Mid Morning	GRAINS	1	4 Vita-Weat crackers	Vita-Weat crackers topped with peanut/almond paste.
	FATS	2	1 tablespoon nut paste eg. peanut or almond	
Lunch	GRAINS	1	1 slice grainy bread	Open chicken sandwich: Top toasted bread with shredded chicken, avocado, tomato and cheese. Grill until cheese is melted.
	PROTEIN	½	50g shredded chicken	
	FATS	1	1/8 avocado	
	MILK	½	20g cheese	
	VEG		Tomato	
Mid Afternoon				
Dinner	PROTEIN	1	6 king prawns	Teriyaki prawn stir-fry: Toss prawns through teriyaki marinade. Stir-fry with finely sliced vegetables of choice. Serve with steamed rice.
	VEG		Non starchy vegetables of choice such as carrot, cabbage, sugar snap peas, snow peas, capsicum, bean shoots or boy choy.	
	GRAINS	1	1/3 cup cooked rice	
	FLAVOUR		Teriyaki marinade	
Evening Snack	MILK	1	200g yoghurt	Yoghurt

1,200 Calorie Meal Plan: Day 5

MEAL	FOOD GROUP	SERVE/S	FOOD CHOICE	MEAL IDEA
Breakfast	GRAINS	1	1½ Weet-Bix	Weet-Bix topped with milk and fruit.
	MILK	1	1 cup milk	
	FRUIT	½	¼ cup tinned or stewed fruit in natural juice	
Mid Morning				
Lunch	PROTEIN	½	50g sliced lean beef	Roast beef and potato salad: Combine sliced cooked potato, blanched green beans, finely sliced red onion and parsley. Top with sliced beef and dress with olive oil and mustard dressing.
	GRAINS	1 ½	1 medium potato	
	VEG		Green beans, red onion and parsley.	
	FATS	1	1 teaspoon olive oil	
	FLAVOUR		1 teaspoon wholegrain mustard	
Mid Afternoon	GRAINS	1	½ cup pretzels	Nut and pretzel mix.
		2	20g unsalted nuts	
Dinner	PROTEIN	1	2 eggs	Spinach, pumpkin and feta self-crusting quiche: Cook onion and pumpkin add spinach. Combine with remaining ingredients and bake in a small ramekin.
	VEG		Onion, pumpkin and spinach.	
	GRAINS	½	1 tablespoon flour	
	MILK	1	30g feta ¼ cup milk	
Evening Snack	MILK	1	200g Greek yoghurt	Berry 'ice-cream': blend yoghurt and berries together.
	FRUIT	½	½ cup frozen mixed berries	

1,200 Calorie Meal Plan: Day 6

MEAL	FOOD GROUP	SERVE/S	FOOD CHOICE	MEAL IDEA
Breakfast	GRAINS	2	2 slices of grainy toast	Open egg sandwich with relish.
	PROTEIN	½	1 egg	
	FLAVOUR		1 teaspoon relish	
	FATS	1	1 teaspoon margarine	
Mid Morning	FRUIT	1	1 medium orange	Fruit
Lunch	GRAINS	1	3 Ryvita crackers	Ryvita topped with ham, cheese, tomato and avocado.
	PROTEIN	½	50g shaved ham	
	MILK	1	40g cheese	
	FATS	2	¼ avocado	
	VEG		Non starchy vegetables/ salad	
Mid Afternoon				
Dinner	PROTEIN	1	100g skinless chicken thigh or tenderloin fillet	Satay chicken with rice and Asian greens: Toss thigh fillets in satay marinade and grill. Steam Asian greens. Serve with steamed rice.
	VEG		Asian green vegetables such as bok choy, broccollini, Chinese cabbage, etc.	
	GRAINS	1	1/3 cup cooked rice	
	FLAVOUR		2 teaspoons satay marinade	
Evening Snack	MILK	1	250ml milk drink	Small latte, cappuccino or flat white OR 1 cup milk with 2 teaspoons milo OR low sugar, low fat flavoured milk.

1,200 Calorie Meal Plan: Day 7

MEAL	FOOD GROUP	SERVE/S	FOOD CHOICE	MEAL IDEA
Breakfast	GRAINS	1	½ cup baked beans	Baked beans topped with grated cheese, a poached egg, sautéed tomatoes and spinach.
	PROTEIN	½	1 egg	
	MILK	½	20g cheese	
	VEG		Tomatoes and spinach.	
Mid Morning	GRAINS	1	4 Vita-Weat crackers	Vita-Weat with sliced tomato.
	VEG		Tomato	
Lunch	GRAINS	1	1 wrap	Cottage cheese, salmon and chive wrap: Top wrap with cottage cheese, salmon, finely chopped chives and shredded lettuce.
	MILK	½	¼ cup cottage cheese	
	VEG		Lettuce and chives.	
Mid Afternoon	FRUIT	1	Apple	Fruit
Dinner	PROTEIN	1	100g lamb	Roast lamb served with baked potato, steamed vegetables, gravy and mint sauce.
	GRAINS	1	1 small sweet potato or potato	
	FATS	1	Oil spray to roast	
	VEG		Non starchy vegetables of your choice.	
	FLAVOUR		1-2 tablespoons gravy 1-2 teaspoons of mint sauce	
Evening Snack	MILK	1	200g yoghurt	Yoghurt sprinkled with nuts or seeds.
	FATS	2	20g nuts or seeds	

1,500 Calorie Meal Plan: Day 1

MEAL	FOOD GROUP	SERVE/S	FOOD CHOICE	MEAL IDEA
Breakfast	GRAINS	2	½ cup untoasted muesli	Muesli topped with milk, yoghurt and fresh fruit.
	MILK	1	125ml milk 100g yoghurt	
	FRUIT	1	2 diced kiwi fruit	
Mid Morning	MILK	½	20g cheese	Carrot and cheese sticks with crackers.
	GRAINS	1	4 Vita-Weat	
	VEG		Carrot	
Lunch	PROTEIN	1	60g tuna 1 hard-boiled egg	Tuna and egg salad: Top shredded lettuce with tuna, egg, parmesan, cherry tomato, green capsicum and jalapenos. Dress with balsamic vinegar.
	MILK	½	20g shaved parmesan	
	VEG		Lettuce, cherry tomatoes and green capsicum.	
	FLAVOUR		Balsamic vinegar Diced jalapenos	
Mid Afternoon	FATS	2	20g almonds	Almonds and apricots.
	FRUIT	1	30g dried apricots	
Dinner	PROTEIN	1	½ cup lean beef mince ½ cup kidney beans	Mexican beef and rice bowl: Sauté onion, garlic, tomato paste, tinned tomatoes, ground spices and beef mince. When cooked, add kidney beans. Top steamed rice with beef mixture, corn kernels, diced cucumber, avocado, coriander, chilli and lime.
	GRAINS	2	1/3 cup steamed basmati rice ½ sweet corn cob	
	FATS	2	¼ avocado	
	VEG		Onion, garlic, tinned tomatoes and cucumber.	
	FLAVOUR		1 teaspoon ground cumin 1 teaspoon ground coriander Lime wedges	
Evening Snack	MILK	1	200g yoghurt	Yoghurt

1,500 Calorie Meal Plan: Day 2

MEAL	FOOD GROUP	SERVE/S	FOOD CHOICE	MEAL IDEA
Breakfast	GRAINS	2	½ cup rolled oats	Porridge with cinnamon and sultanas.
	MILK	1	250ml milk	
	FRUIT	½	3 teaspoons sultanas	
	FLAVOUR		Cinnamon	
Mid Morning	FRUIT	½	1 plum	Fruit and yoghurt.
	MILK	1	200g yoghurt	
Lunch	GRAINS	2	Pita bread	Mediterranean pizza: Top pita bread with relish, cheeses, fresh tomato and pickled vegetables. Grill until cheese has melted.
	MILK	1	20g mozzarella 20g feta cheese	
	VEG		Tomato	
	FLAVOUR		Relish, artichokes, char grilled peppers and Kalamata olives.	
Mid Afternoon	GRAINS	½	2 Vita-Weat crackers	Smashed egg with curry and mayo on crackers.
	PROTEIN	½	1 egg	
	FLAVOUR		Low fat mayo & Curry powder	
Dinner	PROTEIN	1 ½	120g firm white fish 50g prawn meat	Prawn and fish balls: Pulse (gently blend) fish, prawn meat, capers, dill and a squeeze of lemon. Roll into balls, dip in egg wash and breadcrumbs and bake with a drizzle of oil. Serve with tossed salad, avocado and a spoon of tzatziki.
	GRAINS	½	1 tablespoon breadcrumbs	
	FATS	4	¼ avocado 2 teaspoons olive oil	
	VEG		Lettuce, cucumber, tomato and carrot.	
	FLAVOUR		Dill, capers, lemon and tzatziki.	
Evening Snack	FRUIT	1	2 mandarins	Fruit

1,500 Calorie Meal Plan: Day 3

MEAL	FOOD GROUP	SERVE/S	FOOD CHOICE	MEAL IDEA
Breakfast	GRAINS	2	2 slices grainy toast	Cottage cheese and tomato, mushrooms and baby spinach on grainy toast.
	MILK	½	¼ cup cottage cheese	
	VEG		Tomato, mushrooms and baby spinach.	
Mid Morning	MILK	1	250ml milk	Small latte, cappuccino or flat white OR 1 cup milk with 2 teaspoons milo OR low sugar, low fat flavoured milk.
Lunch	GRAINS	1	1/3 cup cooked brown rice	Chicken and brown rice salad: Combine rice, shredded chicken, chopped egg, grated cheese, avocado, cos lettuce, cherry tomato and cucumber. Dress with a squeeze of lemon or lime.
	PROTEIN	1	50g chicken 1 egg	
	MILK	½	20g grated cheese	
	FATS	2	¼ avocado	
	VEG		Cos lettuce, cherry tomato and cucumber.	
Mid Afternoon	FRUIT	1	1 pear	Fruit
Dinner	MILK	1	100g lean lamb steak/ fillet	Lamb fattoush salad: Top shredded cos lettuce with grilled sliced lamb, cucumber, cherry tomato, sliced radish, fresh mint and parsley and torn toasted Lebanese bread. Dress with olive oil and lemon and a spoon of tzatziki.
	GRAINS	2	1 wholemeal Lebanese wrap	
	FATS	2	2 teaspoons olive oil	
	VEG		Cos lettuce, cucumber, cherry tomato and radish.	
	FLAVOUR		Tzatziki, mint and parsley.	
Evening Snack	MILK	1	125ml milk 100g yoghurt	Fruit smoothie
	FRUIT	1	1 cup frozen berries	

1,500 Calorie Meal Plan: Day 4

MEAL	FOOD GROUP	SERVE/S	FOOD CHOICE	MEAL IDEA
Breakfast	GRAINS	2	1 wholegrain English muffin	Smashed avocado, eggs and feta on an English muffin.
	PROTEIN	1	2 eggs	
	MILK	1	40g feta	
	FATS	2	¼ avocado	
Mid Morning	FATS	2	20g almonds (or other nuts)	Nuts
Lunch	GRAINS	1	½ cup Mexican beans	Tomato and bean soup: Sauté onion and garlic. Add canned tomatoes, vegetable stock and Mexican beans. Thinly sliced fresh apple to follow.
	VEG		Onion and canned tomatoes.	
	FLAVOUR		Vegetable stock	
	FRUIT	1	Apple	
Mid Afternoon	MILK	1	40g cheese	Cheese and veggie sticks.
	VEG		Carrot, capsicum or celery sticks.	
Dinner	PROTEIN	1	½ cup chicken mince Egg for binding	Thai chicken burger: Combine mince, cottage cheese, breadcrumbs, curry paste, sweet chili sauce and grated onion. Grill or barbeque. Serve on half a roll with salad.
	MILK	½	¼ cup cottage cheese	
	GRAINS	2	½ wholegrain roll 2 tablespoons breadcrumbs	
	FLAVOUR		Red curry paste Sweet chili sauce	
	VEG		Non starchy salad of your choice such as lettuce, tomato, carrot or cucumber.	
Evening Snack	MILK	½	100g yoghurt	Fruit and yoghurt.
	FRUIT	1	Banana	

1,500 Calorie Meal Plan: Day 5

MEAL	FOOD GROUP	SERVE/S	FOOD CHOICE	MEAL IDEA
Breakfast	GRAINS	2	3 Weet-Bix	Weet-Bix with tinned fruit
	MILK	1	250ml milk	
	FRUIT	1	½ cup tinned fruit in natural juice	
Mid Morning	FRUIT	1	Up to 1 cup strawberries	Strawberry smoothie
	MILK	1	125ml milk 100g yoghurt	
Lunch	PROTEIN	1	½ cup pork mince Egg for binding	Mini pork meat loaf: Combine mince, egg, breadcrumbs, nuts, apple puree and grated onion. Add fennel and caraway seeds and fresh sage if desired. Place mixture in silicon muffin trays and bake.
	GRAINS	½	1 tablespoon breadcrumbs	
	FATS	2	20g pistachio nuts (roughly chopped)	
	VEG		Onion	
	FLAVOUR		2 tablespoons apple puree, fennel and caraway seeds and fresh sage.	
Mid Afternoon	GRAINS	1	½ cup pretzels	Pretzels
Dinner	PROTEIN	1	120g firm white fish	Fish tacos: Bake fish in foil with a squeeze of lime. Add fish to wrap and top with diced tomato, avocado and red onion and drizzle with Coriander Lime Dressing.
	GRAINS	1	1 wrap	
	VEG		Diced tomato and red onion.	
	FLAVOUR		Coriander and Lime Dressing (page 51)	
	FATS	2	¼ avocado	
Evening Snack	GRAINS	½	3 small Salada squares	Cheese on crackers.
	MILK	1	40g cheese	

1,500 Calorie Meal Plan: Day 6

MEAL	FOOD GROUP	SERVE/S	FOOD CHOICE	MEAL IDEA
Breakfast	PROTEIN	1	2 eggs	Breakfast wrap: Whisk two eggs, milk, diced red onion, tomato and spinach. Cook together and serve in a wrap with grated cheese.
	MILK	1	40g grated cheese	
	GRAINS	1	1 wrap	
	VEG		Red onion, tomato and spinach.	
Mid Morning	FRUIT	1	1 apple	Apple spread with nut paste.
	FATS	2	2 teaspoons nut paste eg. peanut or almond	
Lunch	PROTEIN	½	50g shredded chicken	Waldorf chicken wrap: Combine chicken, yoghurt, apple, cucumber, celery, walnuts and smoked paprika. Top wrap with chicken mixture.
	GRAINS	1	1 wrap	
	FRUIT		½ apple diced or grated	
	FATS	2	20g walnuts	
	FLAVOUR		1 -2 tablespoons Greek yoghurt Smoked paprika	
	VEG		Cucumber and celery.	
Mid Afternoon	MILK	1	250ml milk drink	Small latte, cappuccino or flat white OR 1 cup milk with 2 teaspoons milo OR low sugar, low fat flavoured milk.
Dinner	PROTEIN	½	50g casserole beef	Beef and bean hot pot: Sauté diced beef, onions, garlic, celery and carrot. Pour over tinned tomatoes, beef stock and kidney beans and cook slowly until sauce reduces and meat is tender. Serve with mashed sweet potato.
	GRAINS	2	½ cup kidney beans and ½ cup mashed sweet potato	
	VEG		Onions, garlic, celery, carrot and tinned tomatoes.	
Evening Snack	MILK	1	200g yoghurt	Yoghurt topped with berries (fresh or frozen) and muesli.
	FRUIT	1	1 cup berries	
	GRAINS	1	¼ cup muesli	

1,500 Calorie Meal Plan: Day 7

MEAL	FOOD GROUP	SERVE/S	FOOD CHOICE	MEAL IDEA
Breakfast	GRAINS	2	Wholemeal crumpet ½ cup baked beans	Wholemeal crumpet topped with baked beans and grated cheese.
	MILK	½	20g grated cheese	
Mid Morning	MILK	1½	375ml milk	Large latte
Lunch	PROTEIN	½	60g tinned salmon	Salmon cakes: Combine salmon, mashed sweet potato, grated cheese, capers, dill and a squeeze of lemon. Crumb and cook with a little oil in a non stick pan.
	GRAINS	1½	1 egg sized chunk of sweet potato 1 tablespoon breadcrumbs	
	MILK	1	40g grated cheese	
	FATS	2	2 teaspoons oil	
	FLAVOUR		Diced capers, dill and lemon juice.	
Mid Afternoon	FRUIT	1	1 peach	Fruit
Dinner	PROTEIN	1½	100g chicken tenderloins Egg for crumbing	Dukkha crumbed chicken tenderloins and wedges: Coat chicken in egg wash then tip in dukkah and breadcrumbs. Cut potato into wedges, spray with oil. Sprinkle with Moroccan seasoning and bake. Serve with a side salad.
	GRAINS	1½	1 small egg sized potato 1 tablespoon Panko (or regular) breadcrumbs	
	FATS	2	20g Dukkah Oil spray	
	VEG		Non starchy salad of your choice.	
Evening Snack	FRUIT	1	2-3 apricots	Fruit

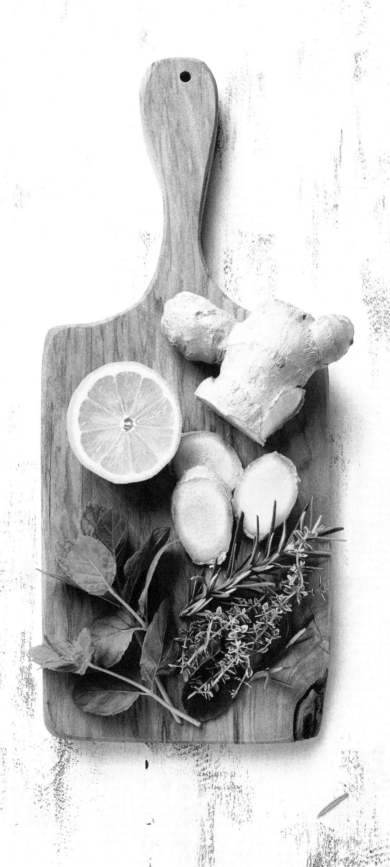

Dressings

Combine all ingredients in a screw top jar and shake well, or add all ingredients to a small jug and whisk until well combined.

MOROCCAN DRESSING

- ¼ cup lemon juice
- 2 tablespoons plain, yoghurt
- 1½ teaspoons honey
- ¼ teaspoon ground cumin
- ¼ teaspoon ground cinnamon
- ¼ teaspoon ground ginger
- Freshly ground black pepper, to taste

VINEGAR BASED DRESSING (VINAIGRETTE)

- 3 tablespoons olive oil
- 2 tablespoons vinegar (white, cider, wine etc. all work well)
- Add black pepper, herbs, mustard etc. as desired

CORIANDER AND LIME DRESSING

- 1/3 cup Greek yoghurt
- 1 tablespoon finely chopped fresh coriander leaves
- 1 tablespoon olive oil
- Fresh squeezed lime juice

Copyright © Nutrition for Weight Loss Surgery 2018

Meal Plan Development: Justine Hawke and Caitlin Davis.
Photography: Shutterstock.
Graphic Design: Jayne Freeman.
Edited by Sally Johnston and Justine Hawke.

www.nfwls.com

CPSIA information can be obtained
at www.ICGtesting.com
Printed in the USA
BVHW050927200421
605396BV00010B/2091

9 780648 664123